PANIC ATTACK

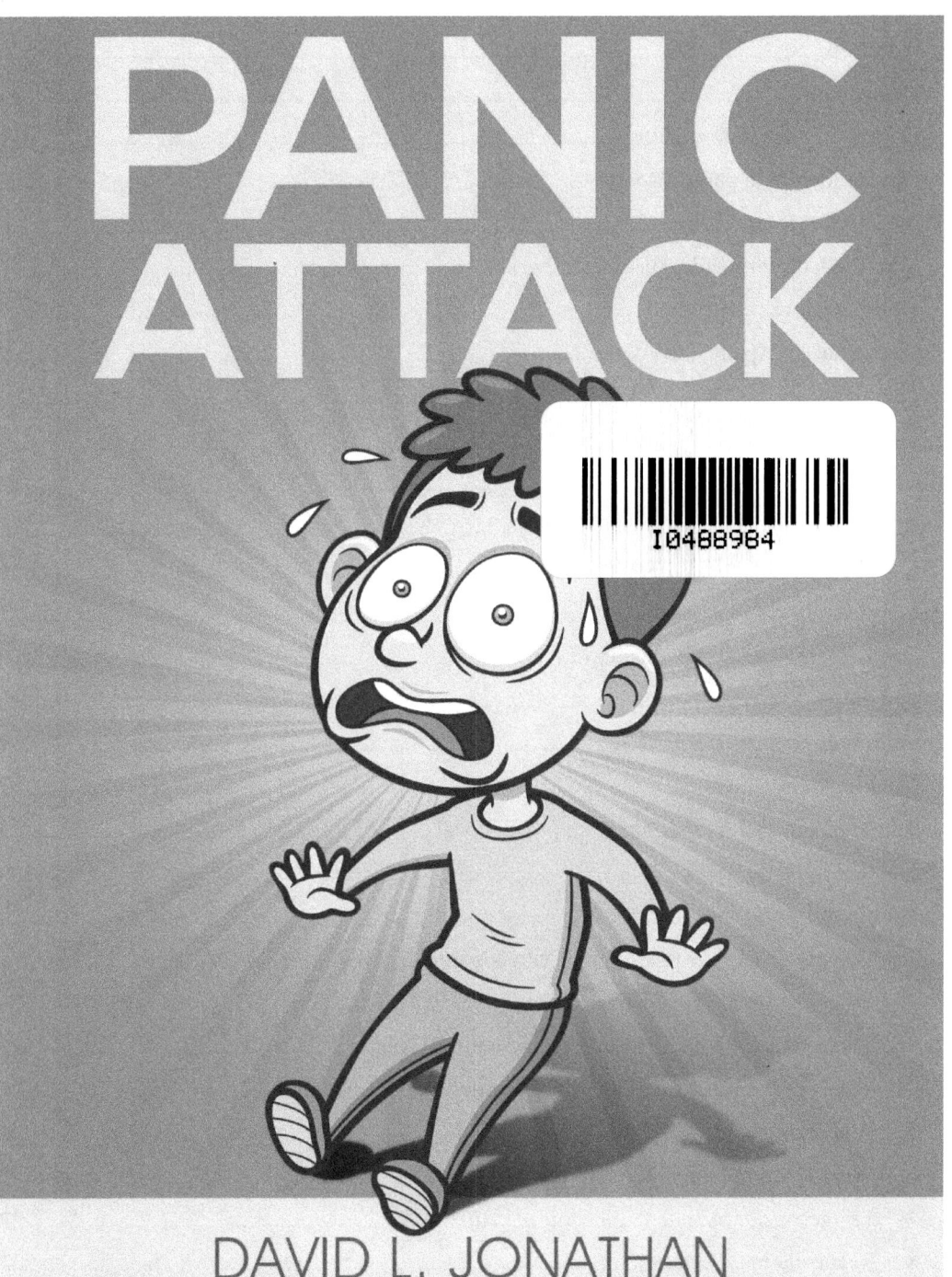

DAVID L. JONATHAN

Contents

What is panic attack

Overview

Presently, due to the major changes in lifestyle, all over the world, people are facing also some sort of psychological issues. Some of them are easily treatable, some other need more time and care to solve. In the following, a brief description of panic attack will be done, in terms of definition, symptoms, causes, treatment (either medical or psychological), ways to prevent panic attacks, and how to deal with it. In conclusion, some other relevant information is available.

In general, the idea of panic attack can be really scary, for the ones having them, as well as the ones having acquaintances with such issues. However, it should be kept in mind these episodes of panic are harmless. The course of a panic attack starts once a person is exposed to some events/happenings, which act like a *trigger*. The attack easily peaks in intensity and also can rapidly go away, with or without help.

The profile of a person facing panic attacks includes different types of fear, such as fear of dying or suffocating. The person might have chest pains or think they have symptoms of a heart attack. Also, they tend to believe of themselves that *are going crazy* and seek to remove themselves from the situation(s) they are in and are provoking this feeling. Together with this feeling, other people may face related physical symptoms. One example is the change in the breathing pace, which increases, or palpitations, that can be described as *hearts are jumping around in their chest*. In addition, they also might feel nausea, smothering sensation, and dizziness. Usually these symptoms fade away in less than an hour.

Studies show that a high percentage of world population has experienced or will experience at least one panic attack during their lifetime. The persons facing these constantly or more than ones should see a specialist in mental health to evaluate their situation. This is because panic attack can be an indication of a panic disorder, depression, or any other type of anxiety based illnesses.

The *anxiety disorders*, briefly said, are the general types of mental-disorder which include panic attacks and some other examples. Anxiety is a normal human emotion, which can be experienced by anyone, at one point or another in their lifetime. A lot of people feel anxious or nervous when they have to face problems at work, or when they take a test, or have to take an important decision. However, the anxiety disorders are different and imply more than just feeling nervous in stressful situations. The difference appears when the anxiety determines such a distress that it strongly affects a person's ability to have a normal life. The types of anxiety disorders include: social anxiety disorder, specific phobias, and generalized anxiety disorder. Not to forget that an anxiety disorder is a serious mental illness. The persons who have anxiety disorders are constantly feeling fear and worry, and this almost prevent them for living their lives.

For example, in United States, the numbers show that many people already are facing full-blown panic attack at least once in their lives, and it usually begins between 15-19 years of age.

A panic attack is even more concerning, because once someone had it at least one time, they become susceptible to develop irrational fears, named phobias, related to the situations when they experienced the panic attack. Further, they develop the tendency to avoid those situations. In time it can become worse, as many people in this situation come to be frightened by doing things that first triggered the panic episode. In the worst case scenario, they become unable to drive, for example, or even step out of the house. In this case, the person is most likely having a panic disorder, associated with agoraphobia.

Panic attacks affect not only a specific category of persons. They tend to appear in adolescents, adults and in younger children as well (even if it is less likely to happen). Adolescents and adults show similar manifestations. Especially the teenagers tend to feel like they are not real, are living in a dreamlike state (derealization), and are frightened of going crazy or dying. In younger children, the symptoms include affections in the ways of thinking (cognitive symptoms). In their case, the panic attacks results in the child's grades declining, decreased school attendance, and avoiding that and other separations from their parents. Children and teenagers with panic disorders present a high risk to develop substance abuse, depression, as well as suicidal thoughts, plans, and/or actions.

Besides panic attack, other anxiety based disorder is the so-called *social anxiety disorder.* Its definition shows that it is the manifestation of an extreme fear to be scrutinized and judged by others in social or performance situations. It should not be mistaken with shyness, as it was inappropriately medicalized.

Also called *social phobia*, the social anxiety disorder can become so extreme that it disrupts daily life. They persons suffering from it usually have few or no social or romantic relationship, they feel powerless, alone, or even ashamed. Some facts about persons in the situation of having social anxiety disorder show the following: (1) about 15 million American adults have it; (2) the typical age of onset is 13 years old; (3) 36% of people with social anxiety disorder report symptoms for 10 or more years before seeking help. People suffering from social anxiety usually admit their fear is excessive and unreasonable, but feel powerless against their anxiety. Moreover, they feel terrified they will humiliate or embarrass themselves. The expression of such a level of anxiety can easily interfere with daily routines, occupational performance, or social life, making it difficult to complete school, interview and get a job, and have friendships and romantic relationships.

Therefore, in terms of anxiety, if someone feels or has sudden attacks of fear that last for several minutes, or if they feel like they have a heart attack/cannot breathe, if these attacks happen at unpredictable times causing worries about the possibility of having another one at any time, then there is a high chance of facing a panic attack.

A *panic disorder* is an anxiety illness, which manifests as sudden and repeated attacks of intense fear, and last for several minutes or even longer, when there is no real danger or apparent cause. They are defined in terms of fear of disaster or of losing control, or fear of dying. In addition, one might have a very strong physical reaction during the attack, which most likely feels like having a heart attack.

The American Psychological Association officially defines *panic attack as a serious condition that around one out of every 75 people might experience. It usually appears during the teens or early adulthood, and while the exact causes are unclear, there does seem to be a connection with major life transitions that are potentially stressful: graduating from college, getting married, having a first child, and so on. There is also some evidence for a genetic predisposition; if a family member has suffered from panic disorder, you have an increased risk of suffering from it yourself, especially during a time in your life that is particularly stressful.*

The panic attack may appear at any moment. This is why many persons suffering from this fear they might have an attack anytime. The triggers of panic attacks are most of the times events or thoughts, which appear for example when taking an elevator or driving. The short list of symptoms – the symptoms are discussed below in detail - include rapid heartbeat, strange chest sensations, and shortness of breath, dizziness, tingling, and anxiousness. Hyperventilation, agitation, and withdrawal are common results. Panic disorder is believed to be due to an abnormal activation of the body's hormonal system, causing a sudden 'fight or flight' response.

In time, those persons suffering from it become discouraged and sometimes feel ashamed because they are incapable of carrying out their normal routines, such as driving, just going to the grocery store, or going to school or at work.

The panic attack usually occurs in the late teens or in early adulthood. Based on gender, it appears more often on women than in men. However, not everyone who experiences panic attacks develops panic disorder.

Many people have just one or two panic attacks in their lifetimes, and the problem goes away, most probably when a stressful situation - the trigger - ends. But if someone had recurrent, unexpected panic attacks and spent long periods in constant fear of another attack, they might have the condition called panic disorder.

Although panic attacks themselves are not life-threatening, they can be frightening and significantly affect the quality of life. However, treatment can be very effective (it usually involves cognitive behavioral therapy, using exposure to reduce the symptoms, and includes medication in some cases).

If the panic attacks are left untreated, they might lead to other problems, such as panic disorder. Further, they might determine individuals to withdraw from their normal activities.

The good news is that panic attacks is curable and the sooner the person seeks for help, the better. With treatment, someone can reduce or eliminate the symptoms of panic attack and regain control of their lives.

Understanding panic attacks

It is important to understand deeper the panic attack, mainly because it does not have very precise features. Of course, there are signs which help recognize it and ask for help, but it is not a very easy thing to do, as there is no clear and precise reason for it. They usually appear out of the blue, without any warning, and may even occur when someone is relaxed or asleep.

Even more, it happens as a one-time experience, but in most of the cases it repeats. Other examples of triggers, besides the ones we mentioned, may be crossing a bridge, or speaking in public. It is that exact situation which determines the person to feel endangered, unable to escape.

A particular description of a panic attack may be in the short story described below:

> *Paula had her first panic attack six months ago. She was in her office preparing for an important work presentation when, suddenly, she felt an intense wave of fear. Then the room started spinning and she felt like she was going to throw up. Her whole body was shaking, she couldn't catch her breath, and her heart was pounding out of her chest. She gripped her desk until the episode passed, but it left her deeply shaken.*

> *Paula had her next panic attack three weeks later, and since then, they've been occurring with increasing frequency. She never knows when or where she'll suffer an attack, but she's afraid of having one in public. Consequently, she's been staying home after work, rather than going out with friends. She also refuses to ride the elevator up to her 12th floor office out of fear of being trapped if she has another panic attack.*

How to identify a panic disorder

It is important to know that usually only a licensed therapist has the knowledge, experience and the ability to diagnose panic disorders. However, the signs that someone should be aware of were already referred to.

Research has showed that sometimes people have to see ten or more doctors before being properly diagnosed, and that only one of four people with the disorder receives the treatment they need. It becomes extremely important, given these numbers, to know the symptoms and to be sure of getting the right help.

Some specialists suggest that if the panic attacks are occasional and if they happened only once or twice, there are not reasons to worry. However, it is a must to keep in mind the key symptom, which is the persistent fear of having future panic attacks. If the attacks repeat (four or more) and there is the fear of having other episodes, this becomes a clear sign to consider finding a mental health professional that specializes in panic or anxiety disorders.

Panic attack symptoms

The American Psychiatric Association's official Diagnostic and Statistical Manual of Mental Disorders defines a panic attack as a discrete period of intense fear, distress, nervousness or discomfort, in which four (or more) of the following symptoms develop abruptly and reach a peak within 10 minutes:

1) Palpitations, pounding heart, or fast heart rate
2) Sweating
3) Trembling and shaking
4) Sensations of shortness of breath or smothering
5) Feelings of choking
6) Chest pain or discomfort
7) Nausea or abdominal distress
8) Feeling dizzy, unsteady, lightheaded, or faint
9) Derealization (feelings of unreality) or depersonalization (being detached from oneself)
10) Fear of losing control or going crazy
11) Fear of dying
12) Paresthesias (numbness or tingling sensations)
13) Chills or hot flashes

The list is even longer, and to keep in mind that sometimes not all of them are present. Therefore, the list of symptoms includes:

1) difficulty breathing, feeling as though you "can't get enough air";
2) terror that is almost paralyzing;
3) dizziness, lightheadedness or nausea
4) trembling, sweating, shaking
5) choking, chest pains
6) tingling in fingers or toes ("pins and needles")
7) fear that you are going to go crazy or are about to die. This is the classic "flight or fight" response that human beings experience when we are in a situation of danger. But during a panic attack, these symptoms seem to rise from out of nowhere. They occur in seemingly harmless situations - they can even happen while you are asleep. it passes in a few minutes; the body cannot sustain the "fight or flight" response for longer than that. However, repeated attacks can continue to recur for hours.
8) it occurs suddenly, without any warning and without any way to stop it.
9) the level of fear is way out of proportion to the actual situation; often, in fact, it's completely unrelated.
10) Sudden and repeated attacks of fear

11) An intense worry about when the next attack will happen

12) A fear or avoidance of places where panic attacks have occurred in the past

A panic attack is not dangerous by itself. It becomes terrifying mainly because it gives the feeling of "crazy" and "out of control". Panic disorder is frightening because of the panic attacks associated with it, and also because it often leads to other complications such as phobias, depression, substance abuse, medical complications, even suicide. Its effects can range from mild word or social impairment to a total inability to face the outside world.

In fact, the phobias that people with panic disorder develop do not come from fears of actual objects or events, but rather from fear of having another attack. In these cases, people will avoid certain objects or situations because they fear that these things will trigger another attack.

Most likely, the majority of the symptoms referred to will show in an episode of panic attack. Therefore, it usually affects the person so much that they become unable to express to others what is happening to them. A doctor is more authorized to note this wide range of symptoms.

A special case of symptoms appear during nocturnal panic attacks, the ones that take place while sleeping. They occur less often than do panic attack during daytime, but affect a large percentage of people who suffer from daytime panic attacks. Individuals with nocturnal panic attacks tend to have more respiratory symptoms associated with panic and have more symptoms of depression and of other psychiatric disorders compared to people who do not have panic attacks at night. Nocturnal panic attacks tend to result in sufferers waking suddenly from sleep in a state of sudden fright or dread for no known reason. As opposed to people with sleep apnea and other sleep disorders, sufferers of nocturnal panic can have all the other symptoms of a panic attack. Although nocturnal panic attacks usually last no more than 10 minutes, it can take much longer for the person to fully recover from the episode.

Recent literature suggests that men and women may experience different symptoms during an attack. Women tend to experience a predominance of respiratory symptoms compared to men.

When to look for medical care

It is important when having a first panic attack to call a doctor's office or the emergency number. The purpose is to be sure that the person's distress is not a heart attack, an asthma problem, endocrine emergency, or other dangerous medical condition.

The medical professional is the only one able to diagnose the panic attack and one should keep in mind there is no such thing as a "wasted" visit to the doctor in this case. Therefore, it is preferred to be told the diagnosis is panic attack than to assume that someone is panicking and be proved wrong.

In almost every case of panic attack's symptoms there is a need of evaluation. If a person who is usually healthy is experiencing a typical attack, they must be shortly and promptly evaluated by a doctor. The level of evaluation depends on many factors.

The medical professionals diagnose the panic attack by exclusion. This means that before the doctor is comfortable with the diagnosis of panic attack, he must first of all consider and rule out all other possible causes.

A typical panic attack can look like many other harmful conditions. Therefore, the doctor must "think of the worst" to be sure not to miss a diagnosis with a potentially more medically serious outcome. In this case the doctor has to take a thorough history and perform a thorough physical examination. More precisely, the doctor is interested in the person's past medical history, past history of any mental illness, and any surgery the person may have had. In addition to exploring whether the person suffers from any other mental illness, the practitioner often explores whether the panic attack sufferer has a specific anxiety disorder in addition to or instead of panic disorder, like post-traumatic stress disorder (PTSD), phobias, obsessive compulsive disorder, or generalized anxiety disorder. Also, the doctor shall ask the patient about medication the person is taking or has recently taken and in what dosage. Moreover, the health-care professional should usually ask about any specific life stress the person may be experiencing.

The list of things that the doctor asks/does before diagnosing, comprise details and information about:

1. Whether panic or anxiety illnesses "run in the family" and about any recent use of alcohol or other drugs by the person. It is important to keep in mind that during the evaluation for an illness is not the time to be untruthful about drug or alcohol habits because both of these factors are critical in the evaluation;
2. About caffeine intake and any over-the-counter or herbal medicines taken;
3. A physical exam will generally consist of a head-to-toe check of all the vital organ systems. The doctor will listen to the heart and lungs and may perform a brief neurologic exam designed to make sure the brain is functioning properly.
4. The doctor will use his or her best judgment regarding the necessity of ordering tests. Given the nature of the symptoms in a panic attack, the person will usually receive an ECG or heart tracing.
5. If the doctor is concerned that the symptoms might be caused by a medical disorder, blood tests, urine tests, drug screens, and even X-rays or CT scans might be ordered.

Moreover, if the person who may suffer of panic disorder/attack has a family history of seizures or symptoms that are not typical for panic attack, a neurologist may be asked to evaluate the person. The reason for this is that some symptoms of panic attack are similar to the symptoms of "partial seizures". Distinguishing between the two is important because the treatment for each is quite different. A neurologist, if consulted, will order an EEG (electroencephalogram) to check for seizure activity in the brain. This is a painless test but does require some time to complete (typically overnight).

When facing symptoms of panic attack, it is important to also now that they often strike when the person is away from home, but also can happen anywhere and at any time. The signs and symptoms of a panic attack develop abruptly and usually reach their peak within 10 minutes. Most panic attacks end within 20 to 30 minutes, and they rarely last more than an hour.

Heart attack vs. Panic attack

Most of the symptoms of a panic attack are physical, and many times these symptoms are so severe that people think they are having a heart attack. In fact, many people suffering from panic attacks make repeated trips to the doctor or the emergency room in an attempt to get treatment for what they believe is a life-threatening medical problem. While it is important to rule out possible medical causes of symptoms such as chest pain, heart palpitations, or difficulty breathing, it is often panic that is overlooked as a potential cause—not the other way around.

Panic attack vs. panic disorder

Many people experience panic attacks without further episodes or complications. There is little reason to worry if a person just one or two panic attacks. However, some people who have experienced panic attacks go on to develop panic disorder. Panic disorder is defined by repeated panic attacks, combined with major changes in behavior or persistent anxiety over having further attacks.

Panic disorder

The symptoms of panic disorder, in addition to what was said before about panic attacks symptoms. The following show that the panic attack already developed into a panic disorder:

1. Experience frequent, unexpected panic attacks that are not triggered by a specific situation, thought, event;
2. The person worries a lot about having another panic attack;
3. The persons are behaving differently because of the panic attacks, such as avoiding places where they have previously panicked.

However, one single panic attack may only last a few minutes, but its effects as an experience leave long lasting mark. When a person has a panic disorder, the recurrent panic attacks take an emotional toll.

The memory of the intense fear and terror that the human being felt during the attacks can negatively impact their self-confidence and cause serious disruption to their everyday life. Eventually, this leads to the following panic disorder symptoms:

1. **Anticipatory anxiety** – Instead of feeling relaxed and like themselves in between panic attacks, the persons feel anxious and tense. This anxiety stems from a fear of having future panic attacks. This "fear of fear" is present most of the time, and can be extremely disabling.

2. **Phobic avoidance** – the person begins to avoid certain situations or environments. This avoidance may be based on the belief that the situation they are avoiding caused a previous panic attack. Or they may avoid places where escape would be difficult or help would be unavailable if they had a panic attack. Taken to its extreme, phobic avoidance becomes *agoraphobia*.

Panic disorder vs agoraphobia

Agoraphobia was traditionally thought to involve a fear of public places and open spaces. However, it is now believed that agoraphobia develops as a complication of panic attacks. With agoraphobia, the person is afraid of having a panic attack in a situation where escape would be difficult or embarrassing. They may also be afraid of having a panic attack where they would not be able to get help.

Given these fears, the persons start to avoid more and more situations. They begin to avoid crowded places such as shopping malls or sports arenas. They also avoid cars, airplanes, subways, and other forms of travel. In the most severe cases, they might only feel safe at home.

A person who is developing agoraphobia usually avoids the following situations:

1. Being far away from home
2. Going anywhere without the company of a "safe" person
3. Physical exertion (because of the belief that it could trigger a panic attack)
4. Going to places where escape is not readily available (e.g. restaurants, theaters, stores, public transportation)
5. Driving
6. Places where it would be embarrassing to have a panic attack, such as a social gathering
7. Eating or drinking anything that could possibly provoke panic (such as alcohol, caffeine, or certain foods or medications)

Although agoraphobia can develop at any point, it usually appears within a year of the first recurrent panic attacks.

Causes of panic attacks

Panic attacks, as a specific type of behavioral illness, is determined by a wide range of causes. There is evidence that sometimes panic attacks are inherited. However, there is also proof that panic may be a learned response and that the attacks can be initiated in otherwise healthy people simply given the right set of circumstances. Research into the causes of panic attacks is ongoing.

In terms of defining the causes of panic attack, it is worth mentioning that panic disorder is a separate but related diagnosis to panic attack.

People experiencing repeated panic attacks and who meet other diagnostic criteria may be diagnosed with this illness. Panic disorder is thought to have more of an inherited component than panic attacks that are not a part of panic disorder. Certain medical conditions, like asthma and heart disease, as well as certain medications, like steroids and some asthma medications, can cause anxiety attacks as a symptom or side effect. As individuals with panic disorder are at higher risk of having a heart-valve abnormality called mitral valve prolapse (MVP), that should be evaluated by a doctor since MVP may indicate that specific precautions be taken when the person is treated for a dental problem.

Research is inconsistent as to whether nutritional deficiencies (for example, zinc or magnesium deficiency) may be risk factors for panic disorder. While food additives like aspartame, alone or in combination with food dyes, are suspected to play a role in the development of panic attacks in some people, it has not been confirmed by research so far.

Anyway, panic disorder sometimes runs in families, but no one knows for sure why some people have it, while others do not. Researchers have found that several parts of the brain are involved in fear and anxiety. Some researchers think that people with panic disorder misinterpret harmless bodily sensations as threats. Researchers are also looking for ways in which stress and environmental factors may play a role.

Nevertheless, one cannot say what are the exact causes of a panic attack or a panic disorder, but the following factor usually play a major role:

1. Genetics
2. Major stress
3. Temperament that is more sensitive to stress or prone to negative emotions
4. Certain changes in the way parts of the brain function

Panic attacks may start off by coming on suddenly and without warning, but over time, they are usually triggered by certain situations. Some research show that the body's natural fight-or-flight response to danger is involved in panic attacks.

For example, if a grizzly bear came after a person, the person's body would react instinctively. The heart rate and breathing would speed up as their body prepared itself for a life-threatening situation. Many of the same reactions occur in a panic attack. However, it is not known why a panic attack occurs when there is no obvious danger present.

Panic attacks can also be caused by medical conditions and other physical causes. In this cases, a doctor must be seen, in order to rule out the following possibilities:

1. Mitral valve prolapse, a minor cardiac problem that occurs when one of the heart's valves does not close correctly
2. Hyperthyroidism (overactive thyroid gland)
3. Hypoglycemia (low blood sugar)
4. Stimulant use (amphetamines, cocaine, caffeine)
5. Medication withdrawal

In other words, the causes of panic attack might come from the body, from the mind or from both.

(Body) There may be a genetic predisposition to anxiety disorders; some sufferers report that a family member has or had a panic disorder or some other emotional disorder such as depression. Studies with twins have confirmed the possibility of "genetic inheritance" of the disorder. Panic Disorder could also be due to a biological malfunction, although a specific biological marker has yet to be identified.

Note: All ethnic groups are vulnerable to panic disorder. For unknown reasons, women are twice as likely to get the disorder as men.

(Mind) Stressful life events can trigger panic disorders. One association that has been noted is that of a recent loss or separation. Some researchers compared the "life stressor" to a thermostat; that is, when stresses lower your resistance, the underlying physical predisposition kicks in and triggers an attack.

(Both) Physical and psychological causes of panic disorder work together. Although initially attacks may come out of the blue, eventually the sufferer may actually help bring them on by responding to physical symptoms of an attack.

(Example) If a person with panic disorder experiences a racing heartbeat caused by drinking coffee, exercising, or taking a certain medication, they might interpret this as a symptom of an attack and, because of their anxiety, actually bring on the attack. On the other hand, coffee, exercise, and certain medications sometimes do, in fact, cause panic attacks. One of the most frustrating things for the panic sufferer is never knowing how to isolate the different triggers of an attack. This is why the right therapy for panic disorder focuses on all aspects - physical, psychological, and physiological - of the disorder.

When discussing about panic attack, other factors should be considered, in terms of risks that might increase the possibility of its occurrence. These include:

1. Family history of panic attacks or panic disorder
2. Major life stress, such as the death or serious illness of a loved one
3. A traumatic event, such as sexual assault or a serious accident
4. Major changes in somebody's life, such as a divorce or the addition of a baby
5. Smoking or excessive caffeine intake
6. History of childhood physical or sexual abuse

Complications

Even if some usually do not go immediately to a doctor, if a panic attack or a panic disorder is left untreated, it can further affect almost aspect of somebody's life. The person may be so afraid of having more panic attack, that they begin to live in a constant state of fear, ruining the quality of their life.

Then, the panic attack develops into complications such as:

1. Development of specific phobias, such as fear of driving or leaving your home
2. Frequent medical care for health concerns and other medical conditions
3. Avoidance of social situations
4. Problems at work or school
5. Depression, anxiety disorder and other psychiatric disorders
6. Increased risk of suicide or suicidal thoughts
7. Alcohol or other substance misuse
8. Financial problems

Treatment

Before taking any medication or doing anything in regard to controlling and treating panic attacks, it is important to firstly see a doctor. As it was said before, the health-care professional is the only one having the expertise to say there is no other physical problem causing the symptoms of a panic attack. Afterward, the doctor may send the patient to a mental health specialist.

In general, panic disorder is treated with psychotherapy, medication, or both.

(Psychotherapy) A type of psychotherapy called cognitive behavioral therapy (CBT) is especially useful for treating panic disorder. The doctor is the only one entitled to recommend this treatment, after diagnosis.

The first part of therapy is largely informational; many people are greatly helped by simply understanding exactly what panic disorder is, and how many others suffer from it.

Many people who suffer from panic disorder are worried that their panic attacks mean they are "going crazy" or that the panic might induce a heart attack. "Cognitive restructuring" (changing one's way of thinking) helps people replace those thoughts with more realistic, positive ways of viewing the attacks.

Cognitive therapy can help the patient identify possible triggers for the attacks. The trigger in an individual case could be something like a thought, a situation, or something as subtle as a slight change in heartbeat. Once the patient understands that the panic attack is separate and independent of the trigger, that trigger begins to lose some of its power to induce an attack.

The behavioral components of the therapy can consist of what one group of clinicians has named "interoceptive exposure." This is similar to the systematic desensitization used to cure phobias, but what it focuses on is exposure to the actual physical sensations that someone experiences during a panic attack.

People with panic disorder are more afraid of the actual attack than they are of specific objects or events; for instance, their "fear of flying" is not that the planes will crash, but that they will have a panic attack in a place, like a plane, where they can't get to help. Others won't drink coffee or go to an overheated room because they're afraid that these might trigger the physical symptoms of a panic attack.

Interoceptive exposure can help them go through the symptoms of an attack (elevated heart rate, hot flashes, sweating, and so on) in a controlled setting, and teach them that these symptoms need not develop into a full-blown attack.

Behavioral therapy is also used to deal with the situational avoidance associated with panic attacks. One very effective treatment for phobias is in vivo exposure, which is in its simplest terms means breaking a fearful situation down into small manageable steps and doing them one at a time until the most difficult level is mastered.

Relaxation techniques can further help someone go through an attack. These techniques include breathing retraining and positive visualization. Some experts have found that people with panic disorder tend to have slightly higher than average breathing rates, learning to slow this can help someone deal with a panic attack and can also prevent future attacks.

Finally, a support group with others who suffer from panic disorder can be very helpful to some people. In is not a replacement for therapy, but it can be a useful addition.

All in all, all of these treatments must be outlined and prescribed by a psychologist or psychiatrist.

 (Medication) Doctors also may prescribe medication to help treat panic disorder. The most commonly prescribed medications for panic disorder are anti-anxiety medications and antidepressants. Anti-anxiety medications are powerful and there are different types. Many types begin working right away, but they generally should not be taken for long periods.

Antidepressants are used to treat depression, but they also are helpful for panic disorder. They may take several weeks to start working. Some of these medications may cause side effects such as headache, nausea, or difficulty sleeping. These side effects are usually not a problem for most people, especially if the dose starts off low and is increased slowly over time. It is important the patient talks to the doctor in case of any side effect.

It is highly important to know that antidepressants can be safe and effective for many people, but they can be risky for others, especially children, teens, and young adults. A "black box"—the most serious type of warning that a prescription drug can have—has been added to the labels of antidepressant medications. These labels warn people that antidepressants may cause some people to have suicidal thoughts or make suicide attempts. Anyone taking antidepressants should be monitored closely, especially when they first start treatment with medications.

The medical treatment for panic attacks may also include **Benzodiazepines**. These are anti-anxiety drugs that act very quickly (usually within 30 minutes to an hour). Taking them during a panic attack provides rapid relief of symptoms. However, benzodiazepines are highly addictive and have serious withdrawal symptoms, so they should be used with caution.

Another type of medication called **beta-blockers** (CBT) can help control some of the physical symptoms of panic disorder such as excessive sweating, a pounding heart, or dizziness. Although beta blockers are not commonly prescribed, they may be helpful in certain situations that bring on a panic attack. Some people do better with CBT, while others do better with medication. Still others do best with a combination of the two. It is also essential to speak with a doctor about any of this medication.

In the process of diagnosis, the doctor might prescribe some other medication, in order to avoid/treat other possible illnesses. Therefore, if the doctor is suspicious of a cardiac (heart) cause, then the person might be given aspirin and various blood pressure medicines.

Once the diagnosis of panic attack is made, however, the person may be surprised that no medicines are prescribed. Before medications are started, the person requires further evaluation by a mental-health professional to check for the presence of other mental-health disorders. These may include anxiety disorders, depression, or panic disorder (a different diagnosis than panic attack).

(**Important**) The person being treated will be closely monitored for the possibility of side effects that can range from minor to severe and can sometimes even be life-threatening. Because of the possible risks to the fetus of a mother being treated with medications for panic attacks, psychotherapy continues to be the treatment of first choice when treatment of this symptom is given during pregnancy.

Psychotherapy is at least as important as medication treatment of panic disorder. In fact, research shows that psychotherapy alone or the combination of medication and psychotherapy treatment are more effective than medications alone in overcoming panic attacks.

Often, a combination of psychotherapy and medications produces good results. Improvement is usually noticed by about three months. Thus, appropriate treatment for panic disorder can prevent panic attacks or at least substantially reduce their severity and frequency, bringing significant relief to up to 90% of people with panic disorder.

Self-Care

It is also possible to deal with panic attack at home, but once again, the person should be careful not to mistake another serious illness (such as a heart attack) for a panic attack. This is a question that many doctors face when people experiencing panic are brought to a hospital's emergency department or the clinic.

All the following recommendations for self-care at home are to be taken just as informative guidelines. In no case there should be the only actions to be taken to treat panic attacks.

(1) caffeine, alcohol, and illicit drugs should be avoided;
(2) one should engage in aerobic exercise and stress-management techniques like deep breathing and yoga on a regular basis, since these activities have also been found to help decrease panic attacks;

A useful technique to overcome symptoms of panic attack (to be read only as tips/recommendation) includes the following steps:

(1) relax the shoulders and become conscious of any tension that you may be feeling in your muscles;
(2) with gentle reassurance, progressively tense and relax all the large muscle groups. Tighten your left leg while taking a deep breath in, for example, hold it, and then release the leg muscles and the breath. Move on to the other leg. Move up the body, one muscle group at a time.
(3) Slow down the breathing. This may best be done by blowing out every breath through pursed lips as if blowing out a candle. Also, place your hands on your stomach to feel the rapidity of your breathing. This may allow you to further control your symptoms.

(4) Tell yourself (or someone else if you are trying this technique with someone) that you are not "going crazy." If you are concerned about not being able to breathe, remember that if you are able to talk, you are able to breathe.

The short list of recommendation and tips of what to do when facing panic attacks issues include:

(1) Learn about panic. Simply knowing more about panic can go a long way towards relieving the distress.
(2) Avoid smoking and caffeine. Smoking and caffeine can provoke panic attacks in people who are susceptible. It is also important to be careful with medications that contain stimulants, such as diet pills and non-drowsy cold medications.
(3) Learn how to control breathing. Hyperventilation brings on many sensations (such as lightheadedness and tightness of the chest) that occur during a panic attack. Deep breathing, on the other hand, can relieve the symptoms of panic.
(4) Practice relaxation techniques. When practiced regularly, activities such as yoga, meditation, and progressive muscle relaxation strengthen the body's relaxation response—the opposite of the stress response involved in anxiety and panic. And not only do these relaxation practices promote relaxation, but they also increase feelings of joy and equanimity.

It is essential to know that if a person is diagnosed with any medical illness, especially heart disease, home treatment is not appropriate. Even if the person has a history of panic attacks, home care is not appropriate if there is any new or otherwise worrisome symptom.

Follow-up
After a person is diagnosed with panic attack, he or she will be given follow-up instructions depending on the entire picture of the illness obtained by the evaluating doctor. Most people are referred for immediate follow-up. Others may be given instructions that follow-up is not needed unless the symptoms return.

Duration of treatment

The success of treatment depends mainly on the patient's desire to attentively follow the recommended treatment plan. Often, it has multiple sides, it will give results in time, not immediately and should start to have noticeable improvement within about 10 to 20 weekly sessions. If the patient continues with the program, within one year there should a tremendous improvement.

Everyone suffering from a panic disorder should be able to find help nearby their homes. It is recommended to seek for a licensed psychologist or other mental health professional, specialized in panic or anxiety disorders. A clinic nearby, with specialists in this domain, it is also desirable. Also, it is important to find the therapist's experience in treating panic disorders.

Nevertheless, panic disorder, like any other emotional disorder, is not something that can be cured by patients alone. An experienced clinical psychologist or psychiatrist is the most qualified person to make this diagnosis, just as he or she is the most qualified to treat this disorder.

The discussion with the health-care professional

Before speaking with a doctor, if possible, the patient should prepare and have details regarding the following:

(1) A list of symptoms, including when the first panic attack occurred and how often happened since then;
(2) Key personal information, including traumatic events from the past and any traumatic events in the past and any stressful, major events that occurred before the first panic attack
(3) Medical information, including other physical or mental health conditions
(4) Medications, vitamins and other supplements and the dosages
(5) Questions to ask the doctor

It is also important to know what to ask the doctor when seeing them for a diagnosis of panic attack. Below it is a list of useful questions to keep in mind. However, it is not exhaustive.

(Ask the doctor)

1. *What do you believe is causing my symptoms?*
2. *Is it possible that an underlying medical problem is causing my symptoms?*
3. *Do I need any diagnostic tests?*
4. *Should I see a mental health specialist?*
5. *Is there anything I can do now to help manage my symptoms?*

(Ask the mental health provider)

1. *Do I have panic attacks or panic disorder?*
2. *What treatment approach do you recommend?*
3. *If you're recommending therapy, how often will I need it and for how long?*
4. *Would group therapy be helpful in my case?*
5. *If you're recommending medications, are there any possible side effects?*
6. *For how long will I need to take medication?*
7. *How will you monitor whether my treatment is working?*
8. *What can I do now to reduce the risk of my panic attacks recurring?*
9. *Are there any self-care steps I can take to help manage my condition?*
10. *Are there any brochures or other printed material that I can have?*
11. *What websites do you recommend?*

(The doctor/mental health provider may ask)

1. *What are your symptoms, and when did they first occur?*
2. *How often do your attacks occur, and how long do they last?*
3. *Does anything in particular seem to trigger an attack?*
4. *How often do you experience fear of another attack?*
5. *Do you avoid locations or experiences that seem to trigger an attack?*
6. *How do your symptoms affect your life, such as school, work and personal relationships?*
7. *Did you experience major stress or a traumatic event shortly before your first panic attack?*
8. *Have you ever experienced major trauma, such as physical or sexual abuse or military battle?*
9. *How would you describe your childhood, including your relationship with your parents?*
10. *Have you or any of your close relatives been diagnosed with a mental health problem, including panic attacks or panic disorder?*
11. *Have you been diagnosed with any medical conditions?*
12. *Do you use caffeine, alcohol or recreational drugs? How often?*
13. *Do you exercise or do other types of regular physical activity?*

(Tests done to diagnose panic attack)

1. A complete physical exam
2. Blood tests to check the thyroid and other possible conditions and tests on the heart, such as an electrocardiogram (ECG or EKG)
3. A psychological evaluation to talk about symptoms, stressful situations, fears or concerns, relationship problems, and other issues affecting the patient life
4. Psychological self-assessment or questionnaire.

(Criteria for diagnosis of panic disorder)

1. Frequent, unexpected panic attacks.
2. At least one of the attacks has been followed by one month or more of ongoing worry about having another attack; continued fear of the consequences of an attack, such as losing control, having a heart attack or "going crazy"; or significantly changing behavior, such as avoiding situations that the patient think may trigger a panic attack.
3. the panic attacks are not caused by drugs or other substance use, a medical condition, or another mental health condition, such as social phobia or obsessive compulsive disorder.

Prevention of panic attack

Panic attack is an illness that once discovered, can be treated, in different ways, and with a lot of tools. However, *panic disorder cannot be prevented.*

The only thing somebody can do is to take a series of action in order to reduce the number of panic attacks with home treatment, and following the recommendations listed above.

In addition, the person should do tension-reducing activities, and lower the amount of stress in their lives. More, they can change the way they think, by Noticing negative thoughts and replacing them with helpful ones. Of course, a balanced diet can only help.

Other factors highly contributing to the lowering of panic attacks occurrences is to stick to the treatment plan and join a support group.

Although it is not a proper prevention of panic attack, in some cases, it can be useful to avoid the stimuli known to trigger the panic attack. This is a valid approach as long as the avoidance does not get in the way of the person's ability to interact with others or otherwise function. For those who go on to be diagnosed with panic disorder or other forms of anxiety, taking the prescribed medications is the key to prevention.

Questions and answers

1. What increases the risk of panic attack/panic disorder?

The risk for panic attacks/panic disorder is higher if:

− Have a family history of panic disorder. You are also at increased risk if you have a parent with either depression or bipolar disorder.
− Have other conditions associated with panic disorder or panic attacks, such as depression.
− Drink alcohol, use illegal drugs, chain-smoke cigarettes, or drink large amounts of coffee or other caffeinated beverages.
− Take medicines known to trigger panic attacks, such as those used to treat asthma or heart problems.
− Have mitral valve prolapse. This is a heart condition in which one of the valves in the heart doesn't close as it should.
− Have had previous, unexpected panic attacks.

2. What is it like to have panic disorder?

"One day, without any warning or reason, I felt terrified. I was so afraid, I thought I was going to die. My heart was pounding and my head was spinning. I would get these feelings every couple of weeks. I thought I was losing my mind."

"The more attacks I had, the more afraid I got. I was always living in fear. I didn't know when I might have another attack. I became so afraid that I didn't want to leave my house."

"My friend saw how afraid I was and told me to call my doctor for help. My doctor told me I was physically healthy but that I have panic disorder. My doctor gave me medicine that helps me feel less afraid. I've also been working with a counselor learning ways to cope with my fear. I had to work hard, but after a few months of medicine and therapy, I'm starting to feel like myself again."

3. Can people with panic disorder have normal lives?

The answer to this is YES, if they receive treatment.

Panic disorder is highly treatable, with a variety of available therapies. These treatments are extremely effective, and most people who have successfully completed treatment can continue to experience situational avoidance or anxiety, and further treatment might be necessary in those cases. Once treated, panic disorder does not lead to any permanent complications.

4. What are the side effects of panic disorder?

Without treatment, panic disorder can have very serious consequences.

The immediate danger with panic disorder is that it can often lead to a phobia. That is because once you have suffered a panic attack, you may start to avoid situations like the one you were in when the attack occurred.

Many people with panic disorder show "situational avoidance" associated with their panic attacks. In worst case scenarios, people with panic disorder develop agoraphobia because they believe that by staying inside, they can avoid all situations that might provoke an attack, or where they might not be able to get help. The fear of an attack is so debilitating, they prefer to spend their lives locked inside their homes.

Even if the person does not develop these extreme phobias, the quality of life can be severely damaged by untreated panic disorder.

A recent study showed that people who suffer from panic disorder:

1. are more prone to alcohol and other drug abuse
2. have greater risk of attempting suicide
3. spend more time in hospital emergency rooms
4. spend less time on hobbies, sports and other satisfying activities
5. tend to be financially dependent on others
6. report feeling emotionally and physically less healthy than non-sufferers
7. are afraid of driving more than a few miles away from home

Panic disorders can also have economic effects. For example, a recent study cited the case of a woman who gave up a $40,000 a year job that required travel for one close to home that only paid $14,000 a year. Other sufferers have reported losing their jobs and having to rely on public assistance or family members.

None of this needs to happen. Panic disorder can be treated successfully, and sufferers can go on to lead full and satisfying lives.

5. *When can/should I call the doctor?*
Call your doctor if you have:

1. Attacks of intense fear or anxiety that seem to come on without a reason.
2. A panic attack or worry that you will have another one, and your worrying interferes with your ability to do your daily activities.
3. Occasional physical symptoms (such as shortness of breath and chest pain), and you are not sure what is causing them.

6. *What symptoms should I consider first?*

It can be hard to tell the difference between the symptoms of a panic attack (such as shortness of breath and chest pain) and the symptoms of a heart attack or another serious medical problem. If you have symptoms of a panic attack, be sure to get medical care right away so that other medical conditions can be ruled out.

7. *Triggers*
If the panic attacks were caused by a specific trigger, such as a medicine reaction, the patient may not need treatment after the trigger has been removed. In this case, that would mean stopping the medicine with the help of the doctor.

But sometimes panic attacks caused by outside factors can continue after the trigger has been removed. They may turn into panic disorder. Panic attacks may also start suddenly without a known trigger.

8. Recurring panic attacks

Even after treatment is stopped because the attacks appear to be under control, attacks can suddenly return. Learn your early warning signs and triggers so you can seek treatment early.

If your panic attacks get too severe or happen too often, you may need to be hospitalized until they are under control. You also may need a brief hospital stay if you have panic attacks along with another health condition, such as agoraphobia or depression. Panic attacks combined with these conditions can be harder to treat.

9. Ongoing treatment

An important part of ongoing treatment is making sure that you are taking your medicine as prescribed. Often people who feel better after using medicine for a period of time may believe they are "cured" and no longer need treatment. But when medicine is stopped, symptoms usually return. So it's important to continue the treatment plan.

You will be continually checked to see if you have other conditions linked with panic disorder, such as depression or problems with drugs or alcohol. These conditions will also need treatment.

10. How can I help a person facing a panic attack?

If someone you know has a panic attack, he or she may become very anxious and not think clearly. You can help the person by doing the following:

1. Stay with the person and keep calm.
2. Offer medicine if the person usually takes it during an attack.
3. Move the person to a quiet place.
4. Don't make assumptions about what the person needs. Ask.
5. Speak to the person in short, simple sentences.
6. Be predictable. Avoid surprises.
7. Help the person focus by asking him or her to repeat a simple, physically tiring task such as raising his or her arms over the head.
8. Help slow the person's breathing by breathing with him or her or by counting slowly to 10.

It is helpful when the person is experiencing a panic attack to say things such as:

1. "You can get through this."
2. "I am proud of you. Good job."
3. "Tell me what you need now."
4. "Concentrate on your breathing. Stay in the present."
5. "It's not the place that is bothering you; it's the thought."
6. "What you are feeling is scary, but it is not dangerous."

By following these simple guidelines, you can:

1. Reduce the amount of stress in this very stressful situation.
2. Prevent the situation from getting worse.
3. Help put some control in a confusing situation.

You can offer ongoing help as the person tries to recover from panic disorder:

1. Allow the person to proceed in therapy at his or her own pace.
2. Be patient and praise all efforts toward recovery, even if the person is not meeting all of the goals.
3. Do not agree to help the person avoid things or situations that cause anxiety
4. Do not panic when the person panics.
5. Remember that it is all right to be concerned and anxious yourself.
6. Accept the current situation, but know that it will not last forever.
7. Remember to take care of yourself.

11. Support for the family

When a person has panic attacks, their entire family is affected. If someone in your family has panic attacks, you may feel frustrated, overworked (because you have to take over his or her responsibilities), or socially isolated because the person restricts family activities. These feelings are common. Family therapy, a type of counseling that involves the entire family, may help.

12. Panic Attacks Prognosis

The prognosis for people who suffer a panic attack is overall, good. Some people have a single attack and are never bothered again. Yet, two-thirds of people experiencing a panic attack go on to be diagnosed with panic disorder. Also, half of those who go through a panic attack might develop clinical depression within the following year, if not treated promptly. Occasionally, a person will, after a long evaluation, be diagnosed with a medical condition that causes panic symptoms.

To keep in mind

1. Seek medical follow-up. For those who are diagnosed with panic disorder, depression, or another form of anxiety disorder, the news is encouraging when treatment is received. These disorders are usually well controlled with medications. However, many people suffer the effects of these illnesses for years before coming to a doctor for evaluation. These conditions can be extremely disabling, so follow-up after the initial visit to the doctor is crucial so that diagnosis and treatment can continue.

2. People who experience panic attacks are not "faking it." They have a real illness. It is important to gain knowledge about the diagnosis to understand and prevent future

attacks. As a person comes to recognize the symptoms of panic attack and complies with whatever treatment is eventually recommended, the person can hope to end the panic attacks.

3. Recent research indicates that adolescents who experience panic attacks are at increased risk for having thoughts about suicide and even for attempting suicide. This underscores the need to receive a thorough evaluation by a doctor.

www.ingramcontent.com/pod-product-compliance
Lightning Source LLC
Chambersburg PA
CBHW071603170526
45166CB00004B/1780